KINESIOLOGY FOR HEALTH

Comprehensive Techniques, Exercises, And Strategies For Optimal Wellness, Pain Relief, And Injury Prevention

DR. MELISSA STOTLER

Copyright © 2023 by Dr. Melissa Stotler

All rights reserved. Except for brief quotations embodied in critical reviews and certain other noncommercial uses permitted by copyright law, no part of this publication may be reproduced, distributed, or transmitted in any form or by any means, Including photocopying, recording, or other electronic or mechanical methods, without the prior written permission of the publisher.

Disclaimer:

The data in this book, is solely meant to be informative and instructional.

This book is not intended to replace expert medical advice, diagnosis, or care. No medical, health, or other professional services are offered by the author, publisher, or any affiliated parties

Individual outcomes may differ in the practice of these therapies, which entail a variety of approaches and methodologies.

A one-on-one session with a trained or certified healthcare professional is still preferable. It is best to consult a trained healthcare provider before making any decisions regarding your health.

The author of this book is not affiliated with any specific website, product, or organization related to any of these therapies.

All reasonable measures have been taken by the author and publisher to guarantee the authenticity and dependability of the material contained in this book.

Contents

CHAPTER ONE 11
  PRINCIPLES OF KINESIOLOGY 11
    Understanding Kinesiological Principles 12
    Key Theories And Models 14
    The Role Of Kinesiology In Health Care 16
    Assessing Movement Patterns 17
    Practical Applications And Examples 19

CHAPTER TWO 21
  ANATOMY AND PHYSIOLOGY FOR KINESIOLOGY 21
    Detailed Muscle Anatomy 22
    Skeletal System Overview 23
    Joint Function And Types 24
    Muscle Contractions And Movements 26
    How Anatomy Affects Movement 27

CHAPTER THREE 29
  BIOMECHANICS IN KINESIOLOGY 29
    Basic Biomechanical Concepts 30
    Analyzing Human Movement 32
    Forces And Their Effects On The Body 33
    Techniques For Measuring Biomechanics 35
    Application Of Biomechanics In Sports 37

CHAPTER FOUR 39
  KINESIOLOGICAL ASSESSMENT TECHNIQUES 39
    Overview Of Assessment Methods 39

    Postural And Gait Analysis 40

    Range Of Motion Testing 41

    Strength And Flexibility Assessments 42

    Interpreting Assessment Results 43

CHAPTER FIVE 45

  KINESIOLOGY FOR INJURY PREVENTION 45

    Understanding The Basics 45

    Common Injuries And Their Causes 46

    Preventative Strategies And Techniques 48

    Role Of Kinesiology In Rehabilitation 50

    Exercises For Injury Prevention 51

    Case Studies And Practical Examples 53

CHAPTER SIX 57

  DESIGNING KINESIOLOGICAL EXERCISE PROGRAMS 57

    Principles Of Exercise Program Design 58

    Developing Goals And Objectives 60

    Structuring Workouts For Different Needs 61

    Incorporating Warm-Ups And Cool-Downs 63

    Monitoring And Adjusting Programs 64

CHAPTER SEVEN 67

  KINESIOLOGY AND SPORTS PERFORMANCE 67

    Enhancing Athletic Performance 69

    Sport-Specific Kinesiological Techniques 71

    Performance Testing And Evaluation 72

    Injury Prevention In Sports 74

    Case Studies Of Athletic Success... 76

CHAPTER EIGHT.. 79

    INTEGRATIVE APPROACHES IN KINESIOLOGY 79

        Combining Kinesiology With Other Therapies 80

        Role Of Psychology In Movement And Performance........................... 81

        Integrative Health Practices 82

        Multidisciplinary Team Approaches... 83

        Benefits Of An Integrated Approach 84

CHAPTER NINE 87

    FUTURE TRENDS IN KINESIOLOGY... 87

        Emerging Technologies And Techniques 88

        Innovations In Kinesiological Research 89

        Potential Career Opportunities.. 92

        Preparing For Advancements In The Field 93

ABOUT THIS BOOK

Kinesiology for Health offers an in-depth exploration of how the principles of kinesiology can transform health care and enhance overall well-being. This comprehensive guide delves into the foundational theories and models of kinesiology, illuminating how these principles apply to real-world health scenarios. Understanding movement patterns and their assessments is crucial for anyone involved in health and fitness, making this book an essential resource for identifying and addressing the nuances of human motion.

An in-depth look at anatomy and physiology reveals the intricate details of muscle anatomy, the skeletal system, and joint functions. This knowledge is pivotal for comprehending how anatomy impacts movement and for applying biomechanical concepts to assess and improve physical performance. The section on biomechanics offers critical insights into human movement analysis, the effects of forces on the body, and practical techniques for measuring biomechanical data. These concepts are fundamental for advancing sports performance and designing effective exercise programs.

The book also provides a thorough examination of kinesiological assessment techniques, essential for evaluating postural alignment, gait, range of motion, strength, and flexibility. Understanding these assessments is key for interpreting results and applying them to injury prevention and rehabilitation strategies. Through detailed case studies and practical examples, readers gain a deeper appreciation of how kinesiology can prevent common injuries and contribute to a robust rehabilitation process.

Kinesiology for Health also addresses the design of exercise programs, emphasizing the principles of goal setting, workout structuring, and the importance of warm-ups and cool-downs. The integration of kinesiology with other therapeutic practices is explored, highlighting the value of a multidisciplinary approach. The book concludes by examining future trends in kinesiology, including emerging technologies and innovations that are shaping the field. This forward-looking perspective is crucial for those preparing for career advancements and seeking to stay ahead in the evolving landscape of health care.

CHAPTER ONE

PRINCIPLES OF KINESIOLOGY

Kinesiology, the study of human movement, rests on several foundational principles that guide how we understand and analyze physical activity. These principles include biomechanics, motor control, and functional anatomy. Each principle plays a crucial role in breaking down the complexities of movement into manageable components.

Biomechanics involves the study of forces and their effects on the body's movements. It examines how forces like gravity, muscle contractions, and external loads interact with our bones and joints. By understanding biomechanics, we can better analyze how movement patterns are generated and how to improve efficiency and reduce injury risk.

Motor Control focuses on how the nervous system coordinates muscle activity to produce smooth and purposeful movements. It involves learning how we plan, initiate, and execute movement. This principle is crucial for designing effective rehabilitation programs and improving athletic performance.

Functional Anatomy is the study of how anatomical structures relate to their functions during movement. This principle helps us understand the roles of different muscles and joints in performing specific actions and how structure variations can impact movement capabilities.

Understanding Kinesiological Principles

To effectively apply kinesiology principles, it's important to grasp their underlying concepts. These principles provide a framework for evaluating and improving movement efficiency and addressing movement disorders.

Force and Motion: In kinesiology, understanding how forces influence motion is key. Forces can be internal, like muscle contractions, or external, like gravity or friction. Analyzing these forces helps in understanding the mechanics behind different movements and the stresses they place on the body.

Muscle Function and Coordination: Muscles work in coordinated groups to perform complex movements. Each muscle has a specific role, whether it's stabilizing a joint or moving. Understanding muscle function and how muscles work together is essential for developing effective exercise and rehabilitation programs.

Postural Control: Maintaining balance and proper posture is fundamental for efficient movement. Postural control involves the interaction between sensory input, motor responses, and the musculoskeletal system. Good posture helps in preventing injuries and enhancing performance in physical activities.

Key Theories And Models

Several theories and models in kinesiology help explain how the body moves and adapts to physical activity. These theories are used to develop strategies for improving movement efficiency and addressing dysfunctions.

The Biomechanical Model: This model explains movement by analyzing the mechanical aspects of human motion. It focuses on forces, torques, and the mechanical properties of tissues. By applying this model, professionals can assess how different forces affect movement and design interventions to enhance performance or reduce injury risk.

The Motor Learning Theory: This theory explores how individuals acquire and refine motor skills through practice and experience. It emphasizes the importance of feedback and practice in improving movement efficiency. Techniques such as task-specific training and feedback are derived from this theory to optimize motor performance.

The Dynamic Systems Theory: This theory views movement as a result of the interaction between multiple systems, including the nervous system, musculoskeletal system, and environmental factors. It highlights how movement patterns emerge from the dynamic interplay of these systems and how changes in one system can influence overall movement.

The Role Of Kinesiology In Health Care

Kinesiology plays a vital role in health care by providing insights into how movement affects overall health and well-being. It helps in preventing, diagnosing, and treating various conditions related to movement and physical activity.

Rehabilitation: Kinesiologists use their knowledge to design rehabilitation programs for individuals recovering from injuries or surgeries.

These programs aim to restore movement, improve function, and reduce pain through targeted exercises and activities.

Preventive Care: By analyzing movement patterns and identifying risk factors for injury, kinesiologists can develop preventive strategies to reduce the likelihood of injuries. This includes designing exercise programs that enhance strength, flexibility, and balance.

Performance Enhancement: Kinesiology is also applied to optimize athletic performance. By understanding the mechanics of movement and muscle function, kinesiologists can develop training programs that improve performance and reduce the risk of overuse injuries.

Assessing Movement Patterns

Assessing movement patterns involves analyzing how an individual moves and identifying any deviations or inefficiencies.

This assessment is crucial for developing effective interventions and improving overall movement quality.

Observation and Analysis: The first step in assessing movement patterns is to observe the individual performing various tasks.

This can include walking, running, or performing specific exercises. Observing these movements helps in identifying any abnormalities or inefficiencies.

Functional Testing: Functional tests are used to evaluate specific aspects of movement, such as strength, flexibility, and coordination. These tests help in identifying areas of weakness or dysfunction that may affect overall movement quality.

Movement Screening: Movement screenings involve evaluating a range of motions and functional tasks to identify potential issues. Common screening tools include the Functional Movement Screen (FMS) and the Performance Oriented Mobility Assessment (POMA). These tools help in pinpointing areas that may require attention.

Practical Applications And Examples

Applying kinesiology principles in practical settings helps in addressing real-world movement challenges and improving overall function. Here are some examples of how these applications can be implemented:

Exercise Prescription: Based on an assessment of movement patterns, exercise programs can be designed to target specific areas of improvement. For example, if an individual has poor core stability, exercises to strengthen the core muscles can be prescribed.

Injury Prevention: Kinesiologists can use their knowledge to develop strategies for preventing injuries. This might include creating warm-up routines that prepare the body for physical activity and recommending proper techniques for lifting or other movements.

Performance Optimization: For athletes, kinesiology principles can be applied to enhance performance. This includes designing sport-specific training programs that improve strength, speed, and agility, and analyzing movement patterns to refine techniques and strategies.

Rehabilitation Programs: In rehabilitation settings, kinesiology principles guide the development of recovery plans. For example, after a knee injury, a kinesiologist might design a program that includes exercises to restore range of motion, strengthen surrounding muscles, and improve functional movement.

By understanding and applying these concepts, individuals can effectively address movement-related issues and improve their overall health and performance.

CHAPTER TWO

ANATOMY AND PHYSIOLOGY FOR KINESIOLOGY

Understanding anatomy and physiology is essential in kinesiology, which focuses on human movement and how it affects overall health. Anatomy refers to the structure of the body and its parts, while physiology explores how these parts function and work together. This foundational knowledge helps in assessing and improving physical performance, diagnosing issues, and designing effective exercise programs.

In kinesiology, you'll delve into how the body's systems interact to facilitate movement. This involves studying how muscles, bones, joints, and nerves collaborate to produce coordinated actions. By mastering these concepts, you can better understand how to optimize physical function and address any limitations or injuries.

Detailed Muscle Anatomy

Muscles are the key players in all movements, and understanding their anatomy is crucial. Muscles are made up of fibers that contract and relax to move. They are typically categorized into three types: skeletal, smooth, and cardiac.

Skeletal muscles are attached to bones and are responsible for voluntary movements. They work in pairs – while one muscle contracts, the other relaxes to allow smooth movement. These muscles have different types of fibers that contribute to endurance, strength, and speed.

Smooth muscles, found in the walls of internal organs like the stomach and intestines, are responsible for involuntary movements, such as those that move food through the digestive system. Cardiac muscle, found only in the heart, is responsible for pumping blood throughout the body. Each type of muscle has a unique structure and function, which is crucial for understanding how the body moves and maintains stability.

Skeletal System Overview

The skeletal system provides the framework for the body and supports and protects vital organs. It consists of 206 bones in adults, categorized into the axial skeleton (skull, vertebral column, and rib cage) and the appendicular skeleton (limbs and girdles).

Bones are not static; they are living tissues that constantly remodel themselves. They are classified by shape: long (e.g., femur), short (e.g., wrist bones), flat (e.g., skull), and irregular (e.g., vertebrae). Each bone type serves different functions, from providing leverage for movement to protecting internal organs.

Joints, where bones meet, are essential for movement. They vary in flexibility and type, including hinge joints (like the knee), ball-and-socket joints (like the shoulder), and pivot joints (like the neck). Understanding the skeletal system's structure helps in diagnosing injuries and designing effective exercise programs.

Joint Function And Types

Joints are the connections between bones that allow for movement and flexibility. They are classified into three main types based on their structure and function: fibrous, cartilaginous, and synovial.

Fibrous Joints: These joints are connected by dense connective tissue and allow little to no movement. Examples include the sutures in the skull.

Cartilaginous Joints: These joints are connected by cartilage and allow limited movement. They are found in places like the spine (intervertebral discs) and the pubic symphysis.

Synovial Joints: These are the most common and movable joints in the body. They are characterized by a fluid-filled joint capsule that allows for a wide range of motion. Synovial joints include hinge joints (elbows and knees), ball-and-socket joints (shoulders and hips), and pivot joints (radioulnar joints).

Each type of joint has a unique structure that supports specific functions, and understanding these differences is crucial for assessing joint health and designing effective movement strategies.

Muscle Contractions And Movements

Muscle contractions are fundamental to all bodily movements and can be classified into several types. Understanding these contractions helps in optimizing exercise routines and rehabilitation strategies.

Isometric Contractions: In this type, the muscle exerts force without changing its length. It's used to maintain posture and stabilize joints.

Isotonic Contractions: These involve a change in muscle length and can be further divided into concentric (muscle shortens) and eccentric (muscle lengthens) contractions. Concentric contractions occur during activities like lifting weights, while eccentric contractions occur during activities like lowering weights.

Isokinetic Contractions: These occur when the muscle changes length at a constant speed, typically achieved with specialized equipment. This type of contraction is used in rehabilitation to measure and improve muscle strength.

Each type of muscle contraction plays a role in different movements and activities, from simple daily tasks to complex athletic performances.

How Anatomy Affects Movement

The way our body moves is directly influenced by its anatomical structure. Each joint, bone, and muscle has a specific role that affects how we perform actions and how efficiently we move.

For example, the range of motion in a joint determines how far a body part can move.

Muscles work in specific patterns to create smooth and controlled movements. The alignment and flexibility of muscles and joints affect overall performance and risk of injury. Understanding these anatomical factors helps in designing targeted exercise programs and making adjustments to improve movement efficiency.

Muscle strength, joint stability, and bone alignment all contribute to our ability to perform various tasks. By studying how these elements interact, kinesiology professionals can better address movement issues, enhance physical performance, and promote overall health.

CHAPTER THREE

BIOMECHANICS IN KINESIOLOGY

Biomechanics is a crucial aspect of kinesiology that examines the principles of mechanics as they apply to human movement.

It involves understanding how muscles, bones, and joints work together to produce motion and maintain stability.

By applying the laws of physics to biological systems, biomechanics helps in analyzing how physical forces affect the body during various activities.

In kinesiology, biomechanics is used to optimize movement efficiency and prevent injury. It encompasses the study of both static and dynamic systems.

Static biomechanics involves analyzing forces on the body when it is at rest, while dynamic biomechanics deals with forces during movement.

By understanding these principles, practitioners can design better rehabilitation programs, improve athletic performance, and enhance overall physical health.

Basic Biomechanical Concepts

Biomechanics relies on several fundamental concepts to describe how forces interact with the human body. These include:

Forces: Forces are pushes or pulls that can cause an object to move or change its motion. In biomechanics, forces are critical in understanding how muscles and joints work together to move.

Levers: The human body acts as a system of levers, where bones serve as levers and muscles provide the force to move them.

Understanding lever systems helps in analyzing how different muscle groups contribute to movement.

Torque: Torque refers to the rotational force around a joint. It plays a significant role in understanding how muscles generate movement around a joint and how this affects overall motion.

Stress and Strain: Stress is the force applied to a structure, while strain is the deformation resulting from that force.

In biomechanics, analyzing stress and strain helps in understanding how different forces impact tissues and joints.

By grasping these basic concepts, one can better comprehend how the body responds to various physical activities and how to optimize movement to enhance performance and prevent injury.

Analyzing Human Movement

Analyzing human movement involves breaking down the complex actions of the body into simpler components to understand how they function together. This process often includes:

Gait Analysis: Studying the pattern of walking or running to identify any abnormalities or inefficiencies. This analysis helps in diagnosing movement disorders and improving athletic performance.

Motion Capture: Using technology to record and analyze movement in three dimensions. Motion capture provides detailed data on how different parts of the body move about each other.

Kinematic Analysis: Examining the motion of the body without considering the forces that cause it. This includes analyzing speed, acceleration, and the range of motion.

Kinetic Analysis: Focusing on the forces that cause movement. This includes studying how forces such as gravity, friction, and muscle contractions affect motion.

By analyzing human movement, practitioners can identify areas of improvement, design effective training and rehabilitation programs, and enhance overall physical performance.

Forces And Their Effects On The Body

Forces have a significant impact on the body, influencing how it moves and functions. Key forces to consider include:

Gravity: The force that pulls objects towards the earth. Gravity affects posture, balance, and the distribution of forces across the body.

Friction: The resistance that occurs when two surfaces interact. Friction impacts movement efficiency and stability, especially in activities like running and jumping.

Muscle Forces: Generated by muscle contractions, these forces drive movement and support the body.

Understanding how muscles generate and apply force helps in optimizing movement and preventing injuries.

External Forces: Forces from external sources, such as weights or resistance bands, that impact the body.

Analyzing these forces helps in designing effective exercise programs and improving performance.

Understanding the effects of these forces on the body is essential for developing strategies to enhance movement efficiency, prevent injuries, and improve overall physical health.

Techniques For Measuring Biomechanics

Several techniques are used to measure biomechanics and analyze how forces and movements affect the body:

Force Plates: Instruments that measure the forces exerted by the body on the ground. They provide data on balance, gait, and the impact of forces during different activities.

Motion Sensors: Devices that track the movement of body segments in real time. They are used in motion capture systems to analyze movement patterns and biomechanics.

Electromyography (EMG): A technique that measures electrical activity in muscles. EMG provides insights into muscle activation patterns and how they relate to movement.

3D Motion Analysis: Using multiple cameras and sensors to capture and analyze movement in three dimensions.

This technique provides detailed information on how different parts of the body move about each other.

By using these techniques, practitioners can gather precise data on biomechanics, allowing for a more detailed analysis of movement and the development of effective interventions.

Application Of Biomechanics In Sports

Biomechanics plays a vital role in sports by helping athletes enhance their performance and reduce the risk of injury. Key applications include:

Performance Optimization: Analyzing how athletes move to identify areas for improvement.

This includes optimizing techniques, improving efficiency, and enhancing overall performance.

Injury Prevention: Understanding how forces and movements contribute to injuries. By analyzing movement patterns, practitioners can develop strategies to prevent common sports injuries.

Rehabilitation: Designing rehabilitation programs based on biomechanical analysis. This helps in recovering from injuries and returning to sports activities safely and effectively.

Equipment Design: Using biomechanics to design sports equipment that enhances performance and reduces injury risk. This includes optimizing footwear, protective gear, and sports apparatus.

By applying biomechanics in sports, practitioners can help athletes achieve their best performance, prevent injuries, and enhance their overall physical capabilities.

CHAPTER FOUR

KINESIOLOGICAL ASSESSMENT TECHNIQUES

Overview Of Assessment Methods

Kinesiological assessment techniques are crucial in evaluating the functional status of the musculoskeletal system.

These methods provide insights into how well the body moves and functions, which is essential for diagnosing issues and planning effective treatment.

The assessment process typically involves a combination of observational and hands-on techniques.

Key methods include postural and gait analysis, range of motion testing, and strength and flexibility assessments. Each technique helps in identifying specific areas of concern and developing a comprehensive understanding of a patient's physical health.

Postural And Gait Analysis

Postural and gait analysis are fundamental components of a kinesiological assessment. Postural analysis involves observing the body's alignment and posture, which can reveal imbalances or deviations that may contribute to discomfort or injury. To conduct a postural analysis, assess the individual from multiple angles—front, side, and back—to identify any misalignments in the spine, shoulders, hips, and knees.

Gait analysis, on the other hand, examines how a person walks or runs. By observing the movement of the feet, legs, and pelvis during walking, you can identify abnormalities such as uneven weight distribution or improper foot placement. This technique often involves using video recordings or specialized equipment to capture detailed gait patterns. Analyzing these patterns helps in diagnosing conditions like overpronation or supination and tailoring appropriate interventions.

Range Of Motion Testing

Range of motion (ROM) testing measures the extent to which a joint can move in its full range. This assessment is critical for identifying restrictions or limitations in joint movement, which can impact overall mobility and functionality. ROM tests are typically performed using a goniometer, a device that measures the angle of joint movement.

During the assessment, the patient is guided through various movements to evaluate the flexibility of specific joints. For example, testing the shoulder may involve raising the arm forward and backward, while hip ROM testing may include leg abduction and rotation. By comparing the measured ranges to normative values, you can determine if there are any deviations from the expected range, which may indicate underlying issues.

Strength And Flexibility Assessments

Strength and flexibility assessments are essential for evaluating the functional capacity of muscles and connective tissues.

Strength assessments measure the ability of muscles to generate force, which is often evaluated using manual muscle testing or dynamometers. Manual muscle testing involves applying resistance while the patient contracts specific muscles, allowing you to gauge their strength and identify any weaknesses.

Flexibility assessments focus on the range of motion and stretchability of muscles and tendons.

Common flexibility tests include the sit-and-reach test, which measures the flexibility of the hamstrings and lower back, and shoulder flexibility tests, which assess the range of motion in the shoulder joint. These assessments help in identifying areas of tightness or reduced flexibility that may affect overall movement and performance.

Interpreting Assessment Results

Interpreting the results of kinesiological assessments requires a comprehensive understanding of normal movement patterns and potential deviations.

After conducting various assessments, analyze the data to identify any patterns or correlations between different findings. For example, a limited range of motion in a joint may be associated with decreased strength or poor posture.

When interpreting the results, consider the individual's overall functional goals and lifestyle. For instance, a runner with limited ankle flexibility might need specific exercises to improve their range of motion and prevent injuries.

Additionally, use the assessment results to track progress over time and adjust treatment plans as needed. Effective interpretation not only helps in diagnosing current issues but also in preventing future problems and enhancing overall physical health.

CHAPTER FIVE

KINESIOLOGY FOR INJURY PREVENTION

Understanding The Basics

Kinesiology, the scientific study of human movement, plays a crucial role in injury prevention.

By analyzing how the body moves and functions, kinesiology helps identify potential weaknesses or imbalances that could lead to injury.

The focus is on optimizing movement patterns, improving strength and flexibility, and educating individuals on how to avoid common pitfalls that may lead to injuries.

Assessment and Analysis

The first step in injury prevention through kinesiology involves a thorough assessment of an individual's movement patterns. This includes evaluating posture, joint alignment, muscle strength, and flexibility. By identifying any abnormalities or imbalances, a kinesiology professional can design a personalized plan to address these issues before they result in injury.

Common Injuries And Their Causes

Muscle Strains

Muscle strains occur when muscles are stretched beyond their capacity, often due to sudden movements or overuse. Common causes include improper warm-up, poor technique, and excessive load on the muscle.

Sprains

Sprains involve the stretching or tearing of ligaments, typically caused by twisting or excessive force.

They often occur in the ankles, knees, or wrists and can result from activities that involve sudden changes in direction or impact.

Joint Dislocations

A joint dislocation happens when the bones in a joint are forced out of their normal positions. This can result from trauma, such as falls or accidents, and can severely impact joint stability and function.

Tendinitis

Tendinitis is the inflammation of tendons, often caused by repetitive stress or overuse. It commonly affects areas like the shoulders, elbows, and knees, leading to pain and reduced mobility.

Preventative Strategies And Techniques

Proper Warm-Up and Cool-Down

A thorough warm-up prepares the muscles and joints for physical activity, increasing blood flow and flexibility.

Similarly, cooling down helps reduce muscle stiffness and aids in recovery. Incorporate dynamic stretches before exercise and static stretches afterward for optimal results.

Strength and Flexibility Training

Incorporating strength and flexibility exercises into your routine helps support and stabilize the body, reducing the risk of injury. Focus on exercises that target major muscle groups and improve joint range of motion.

Strength training should include both upper and lower body exercises, while flexibility training should address all major muscle groups.

Technique and Form

Using proper technique during physical activities is crucial for preventing injuries. Whether lifting weights, running, or participating in sports, ensure that you use the correct form to avoid unnecessary strain on the body. Consider working with a coach or trainer to refine your technique.

Gradual Progression

Avoid jumping into high-intensity workouts or activities too quickly. Gradually increase the intensity, duration, and frequency of your exercise regimen to allow your body to adapt and strengthen over time.

Role Of Kinesiology In Rehabilitation

Assessment and Diagnosis

Kinesiologists play a key role in rehabilitation by assessing the extent of an injury and diagnosing movement-related issues. Their expertise helps in designing tailored rehabilitation programs that address specific needs and promote recovery.

Customized Rehabilitation Programs

Rehabilitation programs created by kinesiologists focus on restoring normal movement patterns, rebuilding strength, and improving flexibility. These programs are customized based on the individual's injury, current condition, and long-term goals.

Monitoring Progress

Regular monitoring of progress is essential to ensure that the rehabilitation program is effective. Kinesiologists track improvements, adjust the program as needed, and provide ongoing support to help individuals return to their optimal function.

Education and Prevention

In addition to rehabilitation, kinesiologists educate individuals on injury prevention strategies to reduce the risk of future injuries. This includes teaching proper techniques, encouraging safe exercise practices, and providing guidance on maintaining overall health and fitness.

Exercises For Injury Prevention

Strengthening Exercises

Strengthening exercises target specific muscle groups to enhance their stability and endurance. For example, squats and lunges strengthen the lower body, while planks and push-ups build core and upper body strength. Incorporate these exercises into your routine to support overall body stability.

Flexibility Exercises

Flexibility exercises, such as static stretching and yoga, improve the range of motion in the joints and reduce muscle tightness. Include stretches for major muscle groups, focusing on areas prone to tightness, such as the hamstrings, quadriceps, and shoulders.

Balance and Coordination Exercises

Balance and coordination exercises help improve proprioception and prevent falls or missteps. Activities like single-leg stands, balance board exercises, and agility drills enhance your body's ability to maintain stability during movement.

Functional Movement Training

Functional movement training involves exercises that mimic everyday activities and sports movements. This type of training helps prepare the body for real-life challenges and reduces the risk of injury by improving movement efficiency and strength.

Case Studies And Practical Examples

Case Study 1: Preventing Lower Back Injuries

A professional dancer was experiencing lower back pain due to repetitive strain. By incorporating a kinesiology-based program focusing on core strengthening and flexibility exercises, the dancer was able to alleviate pain and prevent future injuries.

The program included targeted exercises for the core muscles, stretching routines, and education on proper lifting techniques.

Case Study 2: Shoulder Injury Rehabilitation

An office worker suffered from a shoulder injury due to poor posture and prolonged computer use.

A kinesiologist designed a rehabilitation program that included exercises to improve shoulder stability, strength, and posture.

The worker followed the program diligently, resulting in significant improvement in shoulder function and reduced pain.

Case Study 3: Preventing Ankle Sprains in Athletes

A soccer player experienced frequent ankle sprains. The kinesiologist implemented a preventative strategy that included ankle-strengthening exercises, balance training, and techniques to improve agility. The player reported a decrease in the frequency of ankle injuries and improved performance on the field.

By understanding and applying kinesiology principles, individuals can effectively prevent injuries, enhance their performance, and promote overall health and well-being.

CHAPTER SIX

DESIGNING KINESIOLOGICAL EXERCISE PROGRAMS

Designing kinesiological exercise programs involves creating tailored routines to improve physical function, enhance performance, and prevent injury. Start by assessing the individual's current fitness level, health status, and specific needs. This assessment helps in developing a program that is both effective and safe.

A well-designed exercise program should include a variety of activities that target different muscle groups and fitness components. For example, incorporate aerobic exercises to improve cardiovascular health, strength training to build muscle, flexibility exercises to enhance range of motion, and balance exercises to prevent falls. Each component should be balanced to ensure overall fitness and functional improvement.

Additionally, consider the individual's goals and preferences. A program designed for a competitive athlete will differ significantly from one meant for someone recovering from an injury or looking to improve general fitness. Personalization is key to ensuring adherence and achieving desired outcomes.

Principles Of Exercise Program Design

Effective exercise program design is grounded in several core principles that guide the development of safe and effective routines. These principles include specificity, overload, progression, and recovery.

Specificity means that exercises should be tailored to the specific needs and goals of the individual. For instance, a program for someone aiming to improve their running speed will differ from one designed to enhance upper body strength.

Overload refers to gradually increasing the intensity of exercises to challenge the body and stimulate improvement. This can be achieved by increasing the weight, duration, or frequency of workouts.

Progression involves systematically advancing the difficulty of exercises to continue making gains and avoid plateaus. This principle ensures that the program evolves as the individual's fitness level improves.

Recovery emphasizes the importance of rest and recuperation to allow the body to repair and strengthen. Adequate rest between sessions prevents overtraining and reduces the risk of injury.

Developing Goals And Objectives

Developing clear, measurable goals and objectives is crucial for the success of any exercise program.

Start by identifying what the individual aims to achieve, whether it's weight loss, muscle gain, improved flexibility, or enhanced athletic performance.

Short-term goals are achievable within a few weeks and help build momentum. For example, a short-term goal could be to increase the number of push-ups performed in a set.

Long-term goals extend over several months and require consistent effort. An example might be to run a half-marathon or achieve a specific body composition.

SMART goals are particularly effective. This acronym stands for Specific, Measurable,

Achievable, Relevant, and Time-bound. For instance, a SMART goal could be, "Increase squat strength by 20% over the next three months through a structured strength training program."

Structuring Workouts For Different Needs

Structuring workouts effectively requires understanding the unique needs and goals of the individual. This involves creating a balanced routine that addresses various aspects of fitness.

For general fitness, include a mix of cardiovascular exercises, strength training, and flexibility exercises.

A typical week might consist of three days of cardio (such as jogging or cycling), two days of strength training (focusing on different muscle groups each session), and two days of stretching or yoga.

For weight loss, focus on high-intensity interval training (HIIT) and strength training to boost metabolism and burn calories.

Combining cardio with resistance exercises helps in maintaining muscle mass while losing fat.

For rehabilitation, prioritize low-impact exercises that promote healing without straining the injured area. Gradually introduce resistance training as strength and mobility improve.

For athletes, tailor the program to enhance performance in their specific sport. Incorporate sport-specific drills, agility training, and strength exercises that mimic the movements required in their sport.

Incorporating Warm-Ups And Cool-Downs

Warm-ups and cool-downs are essential components of any exercise program, contributing to overall effectiveness and safety.

Warm-ups prepare the body for physical activity by gradually increasing heart rate and loosening up muscles and joints. Start with 5-10 minutes of light aerobic activity, such as brisk walking or jogging, followed by dynamic stretches that mimic the movements of the workout. For instance, if the workout involves running, include leg swings and high knees in the warm-up.

Cool-downs help the body transition back to a resting state and reduce the risk of muscle soreness. Begin with 5-10 minutes of low-intensity aerobic activity to lower the heart rate gradually. Follow this with static stretches, holding each stretch for 15-30 seconds to improve flexibility and aid recovery.

Monitoring And Adjusting Programs

Monitoring and adjusting exercise programs are critical to ensuring continued progress and preventing injury. Regularly assess the individual's performance, feedback, and any changes in their fitness level or goals.

Tracking progress can be done through various methods, such as fitness assessments, performance tests, or self-reported outcomes. For example, record improvements in strength, endurance, or flexibility to gauge the effectiveness of the program.

Adjustments may be necessary based on progress and feedback. If an individual is experiencing plateauing results or encountering difficulties, modify the intensity, volume, or type of exercise. Adding variety to the workouts can also help maintain motivation and challenge the body in new ways.

Regular evaluations ensure that the program remains aligned with the individual's evolving goals and fitness level, helping to achieve optimal results and sustain long-term adherence.

CHAPTER SEVEN

KINESIOLOGY AND SPORTS PERFORMANCE

Kinesiology, the scientific study of human movement, is crucial for optimizing sports performance. By understanding how muscles, joints, and bones work together, kinesiologists can develop strategies to enhance athletic capabilities.

This field examines biomechanics, motor control, and physiological responses to exercise, providing valuable insights into how to improve efficiency and effectiveness in sports.

Biomechanics: This branch focuses on the mechanical principles of movement. It analyzes forces, lever systems, and joint mechanics to refine athletic techniques. By studying the biomechanics of a soccer kick or a basketball jump, kinesiologists can identify and correct inefficiencies, potentially leading to better performance and reduced injury risk.

Motor Control: Understanding how the nervous system coordinates muscle activity is key to improving sports skills. Kinesiologists assess and train motor patterns to enhance coordination and reaction times.

This can involve exercises that focus on refining movement precision and increasing agility.

Physiological Responses: Athletes need to be aware of how their bodies respond to various forms of exercise and training. Kinesiologists evaluate cardiovascular, respiratory, and muscular responses to optimize training programs. This helps in tailoring conditioning routines that align with the specific demands of the sport.

Enhancing Athletic Performance

Improving athletic performance involves more than just physical training; it requires a holistic approach that includes strength, flexibility, endurance, and mental focus.

Strength Training: Developing muscle strength is essential for performance in almost every sport.

Strength training programs are tailored to target specific muscle groups used in the sport. For instance, sprinters focus on explosive leg strength, while swimmers work on upper body strength to enhance propulsion.

Flexibility and Mobility: Flexibility exercises improve the range of motion in joints, which is crucial for performance and injury prevention.

Mobility drills help athletes maintain fluid and efficient movements. Stretching routines and dynamic warm-ups are integrated into training to ensure that athletes can perform at their best.

Endurance Training: Cardiovascular endurance is important for sustaining high performance throughout a game or race.

Aerobic exercises like running, cycling, or swimming increase stamina and improve overall fitness. Interval training, which alternates between high and low-intensity periods, is often used to mimic the demands of sports.

Mental Focus: Psychological preparedness plays a significant role in sports. Techniques such as visualization, goal setting, and stress management are used to enhance concentration and resilience.

Mental training helps athletes stay focused under pressure and recover from setbacks quickly.

Sport-Specific Kinesiological Techniques

Different sports have unique demands and require tailored kinesiological approaches to maximize performance and prevent injuries.

Running: For runners, kinesiologists analyze gait patterns and running mechanics. Techniques include optimizing stride length and frequency, improving foot strike, and ensuring proper alignment to enhance efficiency and prevent overuse injuries.

Swimming: Swimmers benefit from analyzing stroke techniques and body positioning in the water. Kinesiologists work on improving propulsion and reducing drag by adjusting stroke mechanics and body alignment.

Cycling: In cycling, the focus is on optimizing pedal stroke and bike fit. Techniques include adjusting saddle height, pedal alignment, and body posture to improve power output and reduce strain on joints.

Team Sports: For sports like soccer or basketball, kinesiologists assess movement patterns and agility. They develop drills that enhance quick directional changes, balance, and coordination, which are crucial for performance and injury prevention in these dynamic sports.

Performance Testing And Evaluation

Regular testing and evaluation are essential for tracking progress and making informed decisions about training.

Physical Assessments: These include measuring strength, flexibility, endurance, and cardiovascular fitness. Standardized tests like the vertical jump test, 40-yard dash, and VO2 max test provide benchmarks for performance and help in designing personalized training programs.

Biomechanical Analysis: High-tech equipment, such as motion capture systems and force plates, is used to analyze movement mechanics.

This data helps identify inefficiencies and areas for improvement. For instance, analyzing a tennis player's serve can reveal flaws in technique that impact power and accuracy.

Functional Movement Screening: This method assesses an athlete's ability to perform fundamental movements like squatting, lunging, and jumping. It helps identify any limitations or imbalances that may predispose an athlete to injury.

Progress Monitoring: Regular evaluations track improvements and adjust training plans as needed.

Keeping detailed records of performance metrics and training outcomes ensures that the athlete's program remains effective and aligned with their goals.

Injury Prevention In Sports

Preventing injuries is a critical aspect of maintaining long-term athletic performance.

Warm-Up and Cool-Down: Proper warm-up and cool-down routines prepare the body for exercise and aid in recovery.

Warm-ups increase blood flow to muscles and improve flexibility, reducing the risk of strains and sprains. Cool-downs help in the gradual recovery of heart rate and muscle relaxation.

Strength and Conditioning: A well-rounded strength and conditioning program targets key muscle groups to support joints and reduce injury risk.

For example, strengthening the core muscles enhances stability and protects the lower back during dynamic movements.

Technique Improvement: Proper technique is crucial for preventing injuries. Kinesiologists work with athletes to ensure that movements are performed correctly, reducing the risk of overuse injuries and acute injuries like sprains and strains.

Rest and Recovery: Adequate rest and recovery are essential for injury prevention. Overtraining can lead to fatigue and increase the risk of injury.

Scheduling regular rest days and incorporating recovery techniques, such as massage and stretching, help in maintaining peak performance.

Case Studies Of Athletic Success

Examining real-life examples of athletes who have successfully applied kinesiological principles can provide valuable insights.

Case Study 1: Sprinting Success: A sprinter improved their 100m time by 0.2 seconds through biomechanical analysis and targeted strength training.

Adjustments to their running form and personalized sprint drills led to a more efficient stride and better explosive power.

Case Study 2: Rehabilitation of a Basketball Player: An injured basketball player used a sport-specific kinesiological approach for rehabilitation.

By focusing on functional movement patterns and strengthening the supporting muscles, the player returned to the court with improved stability and reduced risk of re-injury.

Case Study 3: Enhancing Endurance in a Marathon Runner: A marathon runner increased their endurance and race times through a tailored endurance training program. Incorporating interval training and optimizing running mechanics contributed to a significant performance boost.

Case Study 4: Preventing Shoulder Injuries in Swimmers: A swimmer avoided shoulder injuries by implementing a kinesiological approach to technique and strength training. Adjustments to their stroke mechanics and shoulder strengthening exercises improved performance and reduced pain.

These case studies highlight how applying kinesiological principles can lead to measurable improvements in athletic performance and injury prevention.

CHAPTER EIGHT

INTEGRATIVE APPROACHES IN KINESIOLOGY

Integrative approaches in kinesiology involve combining traditional kinesiology methods with other therapeutic practices to enhance overall health and performance.

This holistic view recognizes that human health is influenced by multiple factors, not just physical movement.

By integrating various therapies, practitioners can offer a more comprehensive treatment plan that addresses the body as a whole.

Integrative kinesiology often includes blending physical exercise with techniques such as massage therapy, acupuncture, or nutrition counseling.

This combination aims to address not only the physical aspects of movement but also the emotional and mental components that can impact overall well-being. For instance, integrating mindfulness and relaxation techniques with movement exercises can help reduce stress and improve overall performance.

Combining Kinesiology With Other Therapies

Combining kinesiology with other therapies provides a multidimensional approach to health care. For example, when kinesiology is paired with chiropractic care, it can help optimize alignment and joint function, which enhances movement efficiency and reduces pain. Similarly, when kinesiology is integrated with physical therapy, it supports rehabilitation by focusing on strength, flexibility, and functional movement patterns.

Another common combination is kinesiology and occupational therapy. This pairing helps individuals improve their ability to perform daily activities by addressing both the physical and functional aspects of movement. Integrating these therapies can lead to more effective and personalized treatment plans, ultimately improving patient outcomes.

Role Of Psychology In Movement And Performance

Psychology plays a crucial role in understanding and optimizing movement and performance. Psychological factors such as motivation, anxiety, and mental resilience significantly impact how individuals approach physical activity and rehabilitation. By addressing these psychological aspects, kinesiology practitioners can enhance their clients' overall performance and well-being.

For instance, mental techniques such as visualization and goal-setting can improve athletic performance by helping individuals focus on their objectives and overcome obstacles. Cognitive-behavioral strategies can also assist in managing performance anxiety and enhancing confidence. By incorporating psychological insights into kinesiology practices, practitioners can offer a more holistic approach to achieving optimal movement and performance.

Integrative Health Practices

Integrative health practices combine conventional medical approaches with complementary and alternative therapies to promote overall wellness. These practices acknowledge the interconnectedness of physical, mental, and emotional health, aiming to provide a more comprehensive approach to care.

For example, integrating practices like yoga, meditation, and acupuncture with traditional medical treatments can support the body's natural healing processes and enhance overall well-being. This approach recognizes that health is not just the absence of disease but a state of complete physical, mental, and social well-being. By adopting integrative health practices, individuals can benefit from a more balanced and holistic approach to their health care.

Multidisciplinary Team Approaches

Multidisciplinary team approaches involve collaboration among professionals from various fields to address complex health issues. In the context of kinesiology, this means working with experts from disciplines such as physical therapy, nutrition, psychology, and sports medicine to create a well-rounded treatment plan.

For example, a multidisciplinary team for a patient recovering from an injury might include a kinesiologist, a physical therapist, a dietitian, and a psychologist. Each professional contributes their expertise to address different aspects of the patient's recovery, ensuring that all factors influencing health and performance are considered. This collaborative approach enhances the effectiveness of treatment and supports better outcomes for patients.

Benefits Of An Integrated Approach

An integrated approach to kinesiology offers several benefits, including improved treatment outcomes and enhanced overall well-being. By combining different therapies and addressing various aspects of health, practitioners can create more personalized and effective treatment plans.

One major benefit is the ability to address multiple factors simultaneously, which can lead to faster and more comprehensive recovery. For instance, integrating exercise with nutritional guidance and mental health support can help individuals achieve better results than focusing on one aspect alone.

Additionally, an integrated approach fosters a more holistic understanding of health, leading to more sustainable and long-term improvements in well-being.

CHAPTER NINE

FUTURE TRENDS IN KINESIOLOGY

Kinesiology, the study of human movement, is constantly evolving, and future trends are shaping how we understand and improve human health. As our knowledge of biomechanics, physiology, and motor control expands, we can expect significant changes in how kinesiology is applied in various fields.

One major trend is the increasing integration of technology with kinesiology. Wearable devices and smart sensors are becoming more sophisticated, allowing for real-time monitoring of physical activity and biomechanics. This data helps professionals provide more personalized and precise recommendations for improving performance and preventing injury.

Another key trend is the growing focus on holistic approaches to health. Future kinesiology practices are likely to emphasize the interconnectedness of physical, mental, and emotional well-being. This means that kinesiology will not only address physical movement but also consider factors such as stress management and mental health.

Emerging Technologies And Techniques

Emerging technologies are revolutionizing kinesiology by providing new ways to assess and enhance human movement. Advanced motion capture systems and biomechanical analysis tools are now more accessible, offering detailed insights into movement patterns and forces.

Virtual reality (VR) and augmented reality (AR) are also making their mark in kinesiology.

These technologies can simulate real-life scenarios for training and rehabilitation, allowing individuals to practice movements in a controlled environment. For instance, VR can be used for balance training, while AR can overlay corrective feedback during exercises.

Robotics and exoskeletons are another exciting development. These devices assist with rehabilitation by supporting movement and aiding in the recovery process. They are especially beneficial for individuals with mobility impairments or those recovering from injury.

Innovations In Kinesiological Research

Kinesiological research is continuously advancing, leading to discoveries that enhance our understanding of human movement. Recent innovations include the use of advanced imaging techniques, such as functional MRI and 3D imaging, to study muscle activation and joint mechanics in greater detail.

Genetic research is also contributing to the field. By examining how genetic factors influence movement and susceptibility to injuries, researchers can develop more targeted interventions and preventative measures. This approach helps in creating personalized exercise programs based on an individual's genetic profile.

Additionally, research into the effects of various training modalities, such as high-intensity interval training (HIIT) and resistance training, is providing new insights into how different exercises impact the body. These findings are crucial for optimizing training regimens and improving overall physical performance.

The Role of Kinesiology in Modern Health Care

Kinesiology plays a crucial role in modern health care by bridging the gap between physical therapy, sports medicine, and overall wellness. Kinesiologists work with individuals to enhance movement efficiency, prevent injuries, and aid in rehabilitation.

In clinical settings, kinesiologists assess movement patterns and develop tailored exercise programs to address specific issues, such as chronic pain or post-surgical recovery. They collaborate with other healthcare professionals to create comprehensive treatment plans that address both physical and functional needs.

In sports medicine, kinesiology is essential for optimizing athletic performance and preventing injuries. Kinesiologists analyze athletes' biomechanics, design training programs, and provide injury prevention strategies to help them reach their peak performance while minimizing the risk of injury.

Potential Career Opportunities

The field of kinesiology offers a variety of career opportunities, reflecting its broad applications in health, fitness, and rehabilitation. Some potential career paths include:

Clinical Kinesiologist: Working in rehabilitation centers, focusing on injury recovery and movement optimization.

Sports Performance Specialist: Enhancing athletic performance through biomechanical analysis and tailored training programs.

Fitness Trainer or Coach: Developing exercise programs for individuals or groups to improve overall fitness and health.

Research Scientist: Conducting studies to advance knowledge in human movement and kinesiology.

Ergonomist: Designing work environments and tools to improve efficiency and reduce the risk of injury.

These careers require a strong foundation in kinesiology, but they also offer opportunities to specialize in areas such as sports science, occupational therapy, or rehabilitation.

Preparing For Advancements In The Field

As kinesiology continues to evolve, preparing for advancements involves staying informed and adapting to new developments. Professionals should engage in continuous education and training to keep up with the latest technologies, techniques, and research findings.

Networking with peers and participating in professional organizations can also help. These connections provide access to industry updates, conferences, and workshops that are valuable for professional growth.

Additionally, gaining hands-on experience through internships or research projects can be beneficial. Practical experience not only enhances understanding but also builds skills that are essential for applying innovations effectively in real-world settings.

www.ingramcontent.com/pod-product-compliance
Lightning Source LLC
Chambersburg PA
CBHW071837210526
45479CB00001B/182